Through the Fog WORKBOOK:

A Guide to Caring for Loved Ones with Mental Illness

by

Leah DeMarest

ISBN-13: 9798218347291 (paperback)

Through the Fog Workbook: A Guide to Caring for Loved Ones with Mental Illness

Table of Contents

CHAPTER 1

Understanding Mental Illness

Mental illnesses vary greatly. Each has its own set of symptoms, causes, and effects, making them as diverse as their sufferers. Everything from depression, anxiety disorders, eating disorders, to bipolar disorder, schizophrenia, and post-traumatic stress disorder falls under the umbrella of mental illness.

The Biological Aspect

In many cases, mental illnesses are rooted in biology. Some people inherit genes from their parents that make them more susceptible to certain conditions. These predispositions can lead to the development of a mental illness when paired with environmental triggers or stressful life events.

The Psychological Aspect

The core of many mental illnesses lies in the realm of psychology. Unresolved trauma, feelings, and emotions can give rise to various psychological disorders. Yet, it's vital not to oversimplify mental illness as merely an emotional problem. These conditions are much more complex and multi-layered.

The Environmental Aspect

On top of biological and psychological factors, environmental elements often significantly contribute to mental illness. Traumatic life experiences, high stress levels, exposure to violence, neglect or abuse, can all contribute to the development of these conditions.

What mental illness(s) has my loved one been diagnosed with?

Do I truly understand my loved one's diagnosis?

How do I plan to educate myself further on my loved one's diagnosis?

What are the biological aspects of my loved one's mental illness?

What are the psychological aspects of my loved one's mental illness?

What are the environmental aspects of my loved one's mental illness?

____

____

____

____

Mental Illness Stigma

Despite advancements in our collective societal understanding of mental health, stigma remains a prevalent and persistent issue. It's seen in many forms-from inadvertent remarks at dinner tables to more institutionalized prejudices.

Stigma can be broadly categorized into two types: social stigma and self-stigma. Social stigma refers to the prejudiced attitudes others have about mental illness while self-stigma is the internalizing of these negative stereotypes and prejudices by individuals with a mental illness.

Social stigma manifests in various ways. It's not uncommon to encounter people who harbor biases and misconceptions. They may, for instance, view mental illness as a character flaw or sign of weakness. Outdated and unhelpful beliefs perpetuate these stereotypes, leading to discrimination, reluctance to seek help, and delayed treatment for those affected.

Self-stigma, on the other hand, is intimately related to an individual's self-worth and self-esteem. When someone with a mental illness internalizes societal prejudices, they may begin to believe that they are somehow less valuable than others. This can lead to feelings of shame and worthlessness and can substantially derail the healing and recovery process.

What are some misconceptions I have had about mental illness?

____

____

____

____

What are some misconceptions, judgements, or criticisms I have had toward my loved one due to not understanding their mental illness?

____

____

____

____

How can I help to destigmatize mental illness?

____

____

____

____

How can I support my loved one without using stigmatizing words, actions, and beliefs?

____

____

____

____

How can I help others in my loved one's life destigmatize their view of my loved one and mental illness as a whole?

____

____

____

____

CHAPTER 2

Encouraging a Loved One to Seek Help

It is necessary to approach mental health conversations with a blend of humility, love, and un-wavering patience, and always being mindful of the trust that needs to be nurtured. The talks you have today, the space you hold, has the potential to bring about life-altering transformations tomorrow.

What am I feeling right now as I prepare to have this conversation?

____

____

____

____

What worries do I have about this conversation?

____

____

____

____

What coping skills can I utilize for these feelings and worries?

____

____

____

____

Initiate the Conversation

Addressing loved ones' mental health issues may feel daunting. It's normal to fear potentially triggering fragile emotions or eliciting defensive reactions. Yet, communication is crucial in setting foundations for their healing journey. Conversations about mental health break the ice, unveiling the tools and supports needed for recovery.

What concerns do I have for my loved one?

____

____

____

____

What concerns do I want to bring up in this specific conversation?

____

____

____

____

What time of day, week, month is best to have this conversation? Why?

____

____

____

____

What location is best for this conversation? Why? Is it comfortable, private, and free from distractions?

How am I going to stay calm during this conversation (mantra, deep breathing, take a break)?

How can I encourage self-expression from my loved one? What open-ended questions can I ask to allow them to express their thoughts and feelings?

How can I emphasize my loved one's strengths? What concrete examples can I use of their resilience to remind them of times when they've overcome previous challenges?

Overcoming Resistance and Denials

Encouraging a loved one with mental illness to seek assistance can be an overwhelming challenge, particularly when they're resistant or in denial about their condition. It's essential to approach the situation with patience, sensitivity, and understanding, knowing that acceptance is often the first major hurdle in the journey toward mental health.

What resistance or denial tactics might my loved one use?

What will I do or say if they resist or deny my concerns and/or their need for help?

What coping skills can I use for myself if my loved one resists or denies?

What coping skills can I suggest they use if they have big emotions or behaviors during this conversation?

There might also be the need to involve other individuals in the conversation, but choose carefully. Select people who carry the same message of care, concern, and desire to support healing. High-emotion situations can inadvertently escalate if not carefully managed. If I need to involve others, who might I involve?

____

____

____

____

It's crucial to be prepared for the possibility that your loved one may still refuse help. In this situation, establishing boundaries to protect your own mental health becomes paramount. You cannot force someone to accept help, and it's important to acknowledge that your loved one has a right to make decisions about their treatment. What boundaries can I put in place if my loved one continues to refuse help?

____

____

____

____

Real-life stories of others who've sought help and experienced healing can be powerful proof that things can get better. Focus on their ability to regain control and function, emphasizing the potential for them to find joy and satisfaction in life again. Provide stories of inspiration from your loved one's own life where you remember a time when they were successful.

What tangible examples can I provide about how seeking help can benefit them? What stories of success from their own life can I share to inspire them?

____

____

____

____

____

____

CHAPTER 3

Effective Communication Strategies

One of the most potent tools at our disposal is communication. When it comes to mental illness, the significance of communication cannot be overstated. It isn't just about what you say, but how you say it, how well you listen, and the non-verbal cues you convey.

How have I communicated to my loved one with mental illness in the past? Was it effective and beneficial or did it cause arguments and resentment in the relationship?

____

____

____

____

If past conversations have been negative, what can I improve on?

____

____

____

____

If past conversations have been positive, how can I use these communication skills with my loved one today and in future conversations?

____

____

____

____

Understanding the Barrier

In navigating these barriers, it might help to remember that while you are learning to understand your loved one's new reality, they are also trying to come to terms with their experiences. Empathy, love, and patience are essential in ensuring open and effective communication processes.

What are the barriers in communicating with my loved one?

Physical barriers :

____

____

____

____

Psychological barriers :

____

____

____

____

Social barriers :

____

____

____

____

How can I plan for these barriers if they arise prior to the conversation?

____

____

____

____

How can I plan for these barriers if they arise during the conversation?

____

____

____

____

Active Listening

Active listening involves fully focusing on the speaker, not interrupting, and responding thoughtfully rather than reactively. This mindful approach to communication allows us to embrace empathy and validation, opening a genuine connection and understanding between ourselves and our loved ones.

To manage effectively, it helps to be aware of the physical cues that may reveal what's going on beneath the surface. This includes observing body language, facial expressions, and tone of voice, which often convey more truth than spoken words themselves. By paying attention to these subtle signs, we can better understand our loved one's needs and emotional state, fostering an environment of compassion and trust.

Active listening is a skill, and like any skill, it can be improved with practice. Challenge yourself to employ these techniques in your everyday conversations. The more you practice, the more they'll become an integral part of your communication arsenal, thus enhancing your ability to support your loved one.

How am I going to utilize active listening skills in my conversation (i.e. paraphrasing, validating feelings, patience-not rushing answers, etc.)?

____

____

____

____

Non-Verbal Communication

Non-verbal communication refers to the transmission of messages or signals through a non-verbal platform such as eye contact, facial expressions, gestures, posture, and the distance between two individuals. These silent conversations can speak volumes about a person's feelings, attitudes, and intentions.

However, when someone is suffering from a mental illness, their non-verbal communication may be altered or misunderstood. Interpreting these signals correctly can help you better understand and connect with your loved one.

Do I know my loved one's nonverbal cues (i.e. pacing when they get agitated, lack of eye contact when they are sad, moving their hands when they are anxious, etc.)?

____

____

____

____

Do I know my nonverbal cues and how can I calm those cues during this conversation to not trigger my loved one?

____

____

____

____

CHAPTER 4

Helping a Loved One with Mental Illness

As a caregiver, you shoulder immense responsibility in assisting with tasks such as ensuring medication compliance and helping with job acquisition and retention. However, this role isn't solely defined by functional support. It also encompasses providing emotional bolstering, becoming a reliable source of solace and validation in the often isolating state of mental illness. This dichotomy, of hands-on assistance and emotional sustenance, is a balancing act, one that requires patience and resilience.

How have I tried to help my loved one in the past?

____

____

____

____

What worked?

____

____

____

____

What didn't work?

____

____

____

____

What do I think my loved one needs help with?

____

____

____

____

Has my loved one expressed to me what they need help with?

____

____

____

____

Does what I think what my loved one needs help with and what they have expressed they need me to help them with match?

____

____

____

____

It is important to ensure that my loved one has input in their mental health care and is given the opportunity to make decisions about their life. How can I do more of what they feel like they need and less of what I feel like they need? (It's important to ensure that what your loved one expresses they need is expressed from a sound mind and not out of resentment towards the caregiver, irrational thinking, or psychosis)

____

____

____

____

The Role of the Caregiver

As a caregiver, you play a critical role in your loved one's journey towards betterment. That role can include several facets-from emotional support and physical assistance to aiding them with their critical assignments.

The role of a caregiver in mental health can often feel like a balancing act. As caregivers, we want to provide support while respecting our loved ones' autonomy and encouraging them to take an active role in their recovery. This requires a delicate blend of empathy, understanding, and resilience.

How can I encourage them to take an active role in their care?

____

____

____

____

How can I advocate for my loved one (medical care, mental healthcare, housing, insurance, legislation, etc.)?

____

____

____

____

How can I be emotionally available to my loved one?

____
____
____
____

How can I help them maintain their daily routine?

____
____
____
____

How can I help them maintain their independence?

____
____
____
____

How can I manage logistics (transportation, finances, etc)?

____
____
____
____

How can I help bring normalcy in their life?

____
____
____
____

How can I help provide peace, calm, and hope to my loved one?

____

____

____

____

Assistive Tasks for the Caregiver

As a caregiver for a loved one with a mental illness, you'll encounter a wide range of responsibilities. These tasks often include providing physical, emotional, and social support, aiding with treatment compliance, and ensuring a structured, low-stress environment.

What tasks does my loved one need assistance with?

____

____

____

____

What help does my loved one need with medication management?

____

____

____

____

What help does my loved one need with making and keeping appointments?

____

____

____

____

What help does my loved one need with getting and keeping a job?

____

____

____

____

Does my loved one need help with physical assistance due to other health issues?

____

____

____

____

What help does my loved one need with completing household chores?

____

____

____

____

What help does my loved one need with cooking nutritious meals?

____

____

____

____

What help does my loved one need with childcare?

____

____

____

____

Medication Management

When a loved one is living with a mental health disorder, ensuring they take their prescribed medications becomes a significant responsibility. Adherence to medication not only helps manage symptoms, but also plays a pivotal role in their health and well-being.

Do I know what medications my loved one takes? Why they take them? And the Side effects of the medications?

____

____

____

____

How can I help them establish a routine to take their medication? Do they need a med-minder or a medication dispenser? Do they need a professional to administer their medication?

____

____

____

____

What is the contingency plan for missed doses?

____

____

____

____

Helping my loved one to make and keep appointments

Ensuring that your loved one consistently attends medical and therapeutic appointments is a crucial aspect of helping them manage their mental illness. It's more than simply setting a reminder or driving them to the clinic. It involves understanding their resistance, offering support, and encouraging self-reliance.

What tools can we put in place to help them make and keep appointments?

____

____

____

____

Why is it hard for them to make and keep appointments (fear, anxiety, fatigue, transportation, etc.)?

____

____

____

____

Does my loved one prefer or do better with in-person or telehealth appointments?

____

____

____

____

Helping my loved one to obtain and keep a job

One of the crucial steps towards recovery and normalcy for a person with mental illness is finding a job and maintaining it. Not only does it boost their self-esteem, but it also creates a sense of purpose and structure that significantly aids in mental wellness.

Does my loved one want/need more money?

____

____

____

____

If my loved one gets a job will they lose any other financial or mental health benefits?

Is my loved one cognitively, emotionally, and physically ready for a job?

Does my loved one need a job coach or a special employment program? Do they qualify for these services? Can they afford these services? Are these services available in their community? Is there a wait list for these services?

What are my loved ones' barriers to employment (i.e. lack of stamina/fatigue, poor social skills, they don't interview well, they live in a small town with little job opportunities, etc.)

What are my loved one's interests and preferences (i.e. full-time/part-time, work inside or outside, work from home or in the office, is social/introverted, enjoys working on cars, etc).

____

____

____

____

Physical Assistance

When it comes to caring for a loved one with mental illness, providing physical assistance can sometimes be as crucial as offering emotional support. Several aspects, ranging from helping manage their medication and health appointments to aiding in their daily activities, fall under this domain.

What forms of physical assistance does my loved one need?

____

____

____

____

Emotional Support

When a loved one is living with a mental illness, offering emotional support may often be one of the greatest challenges, yet it's also one of the most crucial facets in their journey towards recovery or management of the illness.

How can I emotionally support my loved one?

____

____

____

____

CHAPTER 5

Building a Positive Relationship

To foster a positive relationship with a loved one suffering from mental illness, begin with setting healthy boundaries. These boundaries are critical in maintaining a balance between caring for your loved one and your personal needs. Develop an understanding of their needs; comprehend their experiences, struggles, and emotions. It allows for more concrete support when both emotional and psychological boundaries are clear. Equally important in cultivating a successful relationship is fostering mutual respect and trust. Involve them in shared decision making, communicate honestly, show devout care, and respect their individuality. Remember, maintaining trust is a continual process and should be preserved even during strained periods. Building a positive relationship with a mentally ill loved one demands patience but is instrumental in creating an environment conducive to recovery and healing.

Do I feel like I currently have a positive relationship with my loved one?

____

____

____

____

How could my relationship with my loved one be better?

____

____

____

____

What steps can I take to improve my relationship with my loved one?

____

____

____

____

Setting Healthy Boundaries

Boundaries are guidelines or rules determined by an individual for their self-protection, health, and well-being.

What boundaries do I currently have in place?

____

____

____

____

What is keeping me from making healthy boundaries?

____

____

____

____

What boundaries are needed in my relationship with my loved one?

____

____

____

____

Practice Empathy and Understanding

Empathy is often confused with sympathy, yet they offer different perspectives. While sympathy involves feeling sorry for someone else's distress, empathy involves seeking to understand and share that person's feelings. Embodying empathy means not merely recognizing someone's pain but also connecting with it. Empathy allows us to feel with others, not just for them.

How can I consciously acknowledge my loved ones feelings and validate their experiences.

____

____

____

____

What are my loved ones strengths?

____

____

____

____

What are my loved ones goals?

____

____

____

____

What are my loved ones interests?

____

____

____

____

What is a symptom(s) of their illness my loved one is often discouraged or struggling with?

____

____

____

____

How can I better see the world through the lens of my loved one?

____

____

____

____

Fostering Mutual Respect and Trust

The journey of supporting a loved one with a mental illness is often broad and complex, but one of the most valuable investments you can make is in cultivating a foundation of mutual respect and trust. This gives strength to the relationship and offers a meaningful space for growth, recovery, and resilience.

How do I currently show my loved one respect?

____

____

____

____

How do I currently show my loved one they can trust me?

____

____

____

____

How can I improve the way I show my loved one respect?

____

____

____

____

How can I improve the way I show my loved one they can trust me?

____

____

____

____

How can I show my loved one how to respect me?

____

____

____

____

How can I show my loved one how to gain my trust?

____

____

____

____

How can I be more consistent in my actions?

____

____

____

____

How can I be a cheerleader for my loved one?

____

____

____

____

CHAPTER 6

Coping with Crisis

When dealing with mental illness in a loved one, you'll inevitably find yourself amidst a crisis (a scenario where the person's mental health situation escalates, posing a risk to themselves or those around them). These moments can be terrifying, but it's important to remember that you're not alone, and there are resources available to help. Recognizing the signs of a crisis is your first line of defense. As a caregiver you've gotten intimate with your loved one's behaviors, making you well-equipped to spot changes.

Have I helped my loved one through a crisis in the past? If so, what went well? What could go better in future crisis?

____

____

____

____

Recognizing Signs of Crisis

The ability to recognize signs of a crisis in individuals with mental illness is a vital aspect of offering them the support they need.

What are the symptoms of my loved one's mental illness?

____

____

____

____

What are the signs and symptoms specific to my loved one when they are starting to spiral?

____

____

____

____

What are the signs and symptoms specific to my loved one when they are in crisis?

____

____

____

____

What are things that have helped my loved one in the past when they are starting to spiral?

____

____

____

____

What are things that have helped my loved one in the past when they are in crisis?

____

____

____

____

Responding to Emergencies

The capacity to respond effectively to mental health emergencies can significantly influence the outcome. An emergency could range from a suicidal crisis to a severe anxiety attack. The response should ideally be swift, knowledgeable, and empathetic, aiming to minimize the likelihood of escalation while assuring the person in distress that help is available and they are not alone.

If I can't immediately be with my loved one in crisis, who can I call to be with them so they are not alone (i.e. friends, family, other supports)? What is their contact information?

____

____

____

____

Loved one's primary care physician contact information:

____

____

____

____

Loved one's therapist contact information:

____

____

____

____

Loved one's psychiatrist's contact information:

____

____

____

____

Local mental health crisis team contact:

____

____

____

____

Mental health hospital contact information:

____

____

____

____

Coping skills I can use to calm myself while responding to my loved one's mental health emergency:

____

____

____

____

People who can support me when responding to my loved one's mental health emergency:

____

____

____

____

Dealing with the Aftermath of Crisis

The crisis has passed, and you're left standing amidst its aftermath. It's time for recovery for both you and your loved one and to begin the healing process. This part of the journey can be equally daunting. This part may involve managing symptoms, dealing with the emotional toll, making practical arrangements, and seeking the help you might still need.

Fighting a mental health crisis with a loved one can be a profound experience, layered with complex emotions and questions. You might be feeling a contrast of relief and exhaustion, burdened by uncertainty about what's to come. It's normal to feel this way. Please, don't feel guilty about your feelings, they are natural and justified.

Who is going to contact my loved one's mental health support team to notify them of the crisis? (support team: therapist, psychiatrist, primary care physician, medication management team, etc).

____

____

____

____

Does my loved one need to talk to their medication management team about a medication change?

____

____

____

____

Does my loved one need to move up any mental health appointments so they can get in quicker due to their recent crisis? Who will they see? Who will call to make this appointment change?

Does my loved one need to add a support they are not already utilizing (i.e.support group, therapist, medication aid, etc.)?

Do I need support from a therapist or support group to help with my mental health after this crisis?

CHAPTER 7

Legal and Financial Planning

Understanding the legal rights of the mentally ill empowers caregivers and loved ones to advocate for just treatment, opportunities, and resources. It lies at the heart of ensuring that your loved one receives the respect, care, and treatment they are entitled to.

Do I know the legal rights for the mentally ill in my loved one's state?

____

____

Preparing Financially for Long-Term Care

One part of effectively planning for your loved one's future with a mental illness is understanding how to prepare financially for long-term care. The financial toll can include not only medication and therapy expenses but also other related costs such as caregiver wages, home modifications, and transportation needs. For this reason, laying out a clear, comprehensive financial plan is a necessary step in preparing for the future.

What are the potential long-term implications my loved one's illness will have on their ability to work, live independently, and look after themselves?

____

____

____

____

Get a clear idea of the resources at your disposal.
Do they have a savings account?

____

____

____

____

Do they have insurance coverage?

____

____

____

____

Do they get government assistance?

____

____

____

____

Do they qualify for any government assistance?

____

____

____

____

What resources and treatments does the above resources cover?

____

____

____

____

How long will these resources and/or coverage last? (i.e. Some insurance plans may limit the number of therapy sessions they'll pay for in a year.)

____

____

____

____

What treatment and resources might my loved one need?

____

____

____

____

How much coverage might we need to have for these treatments and resources? How much might we need to save?

____

____

____

____

Do we needed long term care insurance?

____

____

____

____

Should we consider setting up a trust?

____

____

____

____

Does my loved one need a payee?

____

____

____

____

Does my loved one need a legal guardian? (A guardianship is one form of substitute decision-making which is established through a legal proceeding. The court, after finding by clear and convincing evidence that a person is incompetent, may appoint a guardian to manage the person's care.)

____

____

____

____

Do we need a financial planner to help with this? What are some contacts for financial planners in my loved one's community?

____

____

____

____

CHAPTER 8

Unpacking Self Care for Caregivers

As a caregiver, the risk of emotional and physical toll from the consistent demands of this role is very real. How can you efficiently assist someone else if your own reservoir of strength and resilience is drained? Caregiver self-care incorporates the essential elements of rest, nutrition, exercise, and mental rejuvenation. Your wellbeing propels your ability to offer the steadfast support that your loved one requires.

As a caregivers, you often prioritize the needs of your loved one above our own. However, neglecting your personal needs can lead to mental, emotional and physical exhaustion. This is where the concept of self-care takes on paramount importance. Honoring the need for self-care is not selfish or indulgent; it's necessary for our overall health and vitality, and crucial for you to be an effective caregiver in the long run.

Self-care refers to the mindful actions you take to cater to your emotional, physical, mental, and spiritual well-being. These actions can include anything from getting a good night's sleep, having a healthy diet, meditation, exercise, or even taking time out to read a favorite book or watch a movie. The importance of self-care lies in its ability to bolster your resilience and enabling you to navigate through tough times without succumbing to burnout.

Implementing a Self-Care Plan

A good starting point can be setting aside time every day for an activity you enjoy. Whether it's reading, writing, meditating, or painting – these soul-replenishing habits can improve your mood and lower your stress levels over time.

What activity/activities will be my go-to soul-replenishing habits?

____

____

____

____

How often will I fit these activities into my schedule?

____

____

____

____

How can I implement exercise into my regular schedule? What kinds of exercise activities will I do?

____

____

____

____

Is there a certain time of day or day of the week to schedule these activities?

____

____

____

____

Being intentional about specific times that you will do an activity will cause you to be more apt to actually do the activity scheduled. Where will I record these activities (calendar, phone, planner, etc.)?

How can I implement a healthy diet into my life (i.e. limit junk food, what healthy food options will replace my current unhealthy food options, what healthy recipes do I want to try)?

Recipes

How can I improve my sleep habits?

____

____

____

____

What friends or family can I turn to in order to ensure I include fun and laughter into my life? What activities might we do/try?

____

____

____

____

Do I need a therapist or support group?

____

____

____

____

Create an activity bucket list of things you want to do or new things you want to try. Make a point to incorporate these activities into your schedule either weekly, monthly, or quarterly.

What goals do I want to accomplish in my life?

Short-term goals:

Long-term goals:

My positive affirmations list:

CHAPTER 9

Resources and Support

This chapter is an overview of the various outside resources that are available such as mental health professionals, clinics, and support groups tailored for caregivers. Additionally, an array of online resources exist that can help improve your understanding of mental health issues, provide advice for managing crises, and offer platforms for you to connect and share experiences with other caregivers.

Mental Health Professionals and Clinics

Psychiatrists in my loved one's community:

____

____

____

____

Psychologists in my loved one's community:

____

____

____

____

Therapists/counselors in my loved one's community:

____

____

____

____

Mental health clinics in my loved one's community:

____

____

____

____

Residential treatment centers in my loved one's community:

____

____

____

____

Day programs in my loved one's community:

____

____

____

____

Support groups in my loved one's community:

____

____

____

____

Medication management in my loved one's community:

____

____

____

____

Payee services in my loved one's community:

____

____

____

____

Food banks in my loved one's community:

____

____

____

____

Clothing closets in my loved one's community:

____

____

____

____

Social Security benefits office contact information:

____

____

____

____

Medicaid office contact information:

____

____

____

____

Support for Caregivers

Caregiver support groups in my area:

____

____

____

____

Therapist/counselor in my area:

____

____

____

____

Respite care contact information:

____

____

____

____

Online Resources for Mental Health

-psychologytoday.com (help with finding a therapist/counselor or psychiatrist/psychologist)
-Give an Hour program for veterans and/or their families to receive free therapy
-Telemental health therapy
    -teladoc.com
    -amwell.com
    -other:

-Online peer support communities
    -Mental Health America
    -Reddit
    -Elefriends

-Nonprofit organizations and governing bodies
    -American Psychiatric Association (APA)
    -National Alliance on Mental Illness (NAMI)
    -Anxiety and Depression Association of America
    -The Trevor Project (LGBTQ+)
    -American Foundation for Suicide Prevention (AFSP)
    -The Foundation for Post-Traumatic Healing (CPTSD Foundation)
    -National Federation of Families
    -To Write Love on Her Arms (TWLOHA)
    -International OCD Foundations
    -National Institute for Mental Health (NIMH)
    -International Bipolar Foundation
    -National Education Alliance for Borderline Personality Disorder
    -Wounded Warrior Project (veterans)

-Crisis Lines
(There are local crisis hotlines for each state. Below are the national hotlines.)
    -National Mental Health Hotline: 866-903-3787
    -Crisis Text Line: Text 'HOME' to 741741
    -National Suicide and Crisis Lifeline: dial 988
    -Veteran Crisis Lifeline: dial 988, then press 1; Text 838255
    -National Sexual Assault Hotline: 1-800-656-4673
    -National Domestic Violence Hotline: 1-800-799-7233
    -Substance Abuse and Mental Health Services (SAMHSA): 800-662-4357
    -NAMI: Available Monday Through Friday, 10 A.M. – 10 P.M., ET.
    Call 1-800-950-NAMI (6264), text "HelpLine" to 62640 or email us at helpline@nami.org

Further Resources and Activities

Activity 1. Six Areas of Self-Care

It's important to practice self-care in the six main areas of life: physical, psychological, emotional, spiritual, personal, and professional.

Examples of self-care in each area:

Physical: safe housing, regular medical care, healthy eating, exercise, sleep, get a hug, explore physical intimacy.

Psychological: therapy, self-reflection, journaling, aromatherapy, draw, paint, relax in the sun, garden, read a self-help book, positive affirmations, join a support group.

Emotional: laugh, self-love, self-compassion, watch a funny movie, practice forgiveness, find a hobby, positive affirmations, volunteer, cuddle with your pet.

Spiritual: pray, spend time in nature, spend time in your spiritual community, meditate, Bible study, self-reflection.

Personal: plan short and long-term goals, make a vision board, spend time with friends and family, play a musical instrument.

Professional: take time for lunch, take your allotted breaks, set boundaries, leave work at work, do not take overtime, do not work during your time off, learn to say no, take a class, take all of your vacation and sick days, plan your next career move.

How can I practice physical self-care?

____

____

____

____

How can I practice psychological self-care?

____

____

____

____

How can I practice emotional self-care?

How can I practice spiritual self-care?

How can I practice personal self-care?

How can I practice professional self-care?

Activity 2. Realm Of Control

We can control our thoughts, feelings, emotions, behaviors, and reactions. We can not control someone else's thoughts, feelings, emotions, behaviors, and reactions. We can't control the weather, traffic, how much work our supervisor gives us, etc. We can control how we think and feel about these situations and how we react to these situations.

List a negative situation:

____

____

____

____

What can I control about this negative situation?

____

____

____

____

What can't I control about this situation?

____

____

____

____

Activity 3. Reframing Negative Thoughts

Reframing is a technique used to shift your mindset so you're able to look at a situation, person, or relationship from a slightly different perspective. Reframing can be useful for people who are experiencing mental health conditions, but it can also be helpful for improving overall mental well-being. Using reframing can help you become more positive and resilient in the face of life's challenges.

Negative Thought	Reframed Thought
I'm a failure	I'm learning
I will never be able to save money	I can get a financial planner for support
What if I go and have a terrible time	I'll go with my friend who supports me

Activity 4. Feelings Processing

It can be tough to process feelings when going through a difficult time. Sometimes it can even be difficult to identify how you feel about a situation and why, let alone know how to improve the situation. The next time you are having a bad day or struggling with a negative situation, write down a list of all of the feelings you felt throughout the difficult day or that you feel about the negative situation. Next to each feeling write down what made you feel that feeling. Next to the 'what' write down why that made you feel that feeling. And finally, next to the 'why' write down what you can do to improve the situation or how you think or feel about the situation.

Feelings	What made me feel this way	Why did it make me feel this way	What can I do about it
Frustrated	I made a mistake at work	I was embarrassed and worried because I didn't want my boss to think I was incompetent	Improve my skills, ask more questions, and get more training to prevent mistakes in the future

Resource 1. Coping Skills Examples

1. Take deep breaths	42. Ask for help
2. Take a walk	43. Spend time in nature
3. Stretch	44. Mindfulness techniques
4. Yoga	45. Progressive muscle relaxation
5. Listen to music	46. Watch the clouds
6. Take a break	47. Make a scrap book
7. Count to ten	48. Remember realm of control
8. Use positive self-talk	49. Stimulate the vagus nerve
9. Talk to a friend	50. Crafts
10. Take a nap	51. Take a boxing class
11. Visualize a calm place	52. Take a shower or bath
12. Spend time with a pet	53. Get a manicure or pedicure
13. Get a snack	54. Get a facial
14. Read a book	55. Get a massage
15. Go for a jog	56. Cry
16. Ride your bike	57. Yell into a pillow
17. Journal	58. Schedule a smash room
18. Draw	59. Sing
19. Clean	60. Eat healthy food
20. Color	61. Laugh with friends
21. Meditate	62. Spend time with people who love you
22. Use a stress ball	63. Pray
23. Dance	64. Play basketball, soccer, etc.
24. Write a letter	65. Aromatherapy
25. Look at pictures you've taken	66. Use fidget tools
26. Make a gratitude list	67. Do something spiritual
27. List your positive qualities	68. Make a vision board
28. Do something kind	69. Skip rocks
29. Hug	70. Suck on a mint or ice cube
30. Put a puzzle together	71. Watch funny videos
31. Watch a movie	72. Build with legos
32. Play a musical instrument	73. Practice letting go
33. Garden	74. Take a mental health day
34. Take pictures	75. Organize a room or clutter
35. Chew gum	76. Go to a support group
36. Paint your nails	77. Go to a museum or the zoo
37. Read inspirational quotes	78. Get a hair cut
38. Cook or bake	79. Schedule a therapy session
39. Use an 'I statement'	80. Go swimming
40. Identify your emotions	81. Sit in a hot tub
41. Express your feelings to someone	82. Smell candles or flowers

Resource 2. Examples of Positive Affirmations

1.	I am worthy	41.	I am brave
2.	I am powerful	42.	I am whole
3.	I am enough	43.	I am strong
4.	I am competent	44.	I'm working at my own pace
5.	I am intelligent	45.	I'm prepared to succeed
6.	I believe in my abilities	46.	Today I'm going to shine
7.	I am beautiful	47.	I'm important
8.	I can do it	48.	I trust my decisions
9.	I am successful	49.	I am resilient
10.	I am confident	50.	I choose myself
11.	I am loved	51.	I can do hard things
12.	I am proud of...	52.	I overcome my fears
13.	I can face any challenge	53.	I am trustworthy
14.	I believe in myself	54.	I am loving
15.	I am capable	55.	I am compassionate
16.	I can clearly state my needs	56.	I am safe and supported
17.	Today is a great day	57.	I am content
18.	I love myself	58.	I am good at art
19.	I am getting better	59.	I am a skilled cook
20.	I am an unstoppable force	60.	I am good my job
21.	I am inspiring	61.	I am a great friend
22.	I am filled with focus	62.	I am responsible
23.	I am grateful	63.	I breathe in healing and exhale pain
24.	Obstacles are motivation	64.	I celebrate the good qualities
25.	I am learning	65.	I embrace change
26.	I accept myself for who I am	66.	I hold community for others
27.	My life has meaning	67.	I am good at basketball
28.	I accomplished_______ today	68.	I am a good communicator
29.	I am fun	69.	I was productive today by...
30.	All of my problems have solutions	70.	Something that made me happy today is...
31.	Today I am a leader	71.	I love that I am.....
32.	I forgive myself for mistakes	72.	My perspective is unique
33.	I have courage	73.	My weirdness is wonderful
34.	I can control my own happiness	74.	Sometimes the work is resting
35.	I have people who love and respect me	75.	There is growth in stillness
36.	I stand for what I believe in	76.	Something that made me feel confident today was...
37.	I can do better next time	77.	I can be calm
38.	I give myself permission to...	78.	I can control my emotions
39.	I matter		
40.	I only compare myself to myself		